Hospice Patient Visit Notes

Created by Nurses, for Nurses

This Notebook Belongs To:

_____

"I'm a little pencil in the hand of a writing God who is sending a love letter to the world."

- Mother Teresa

Greetings, Fellow Nurses!

The vocation of nursing is a special one. Those of us who choose hospice are especially blessed to serve others during the most important moments of their lives, as well as being present to family and friends.

I am hopeful this notebook will be an assistance to you, especially when you are busy and can't do the 'bedside' charting we all strive to do. Instead of writing vital signs and other info on spare paper or whatever else you might find, this notebook will be a tool to keep all your notes together, for use later when you enter the appropriate info into your EMR.

Please contact me via derekjflores.com with any feedback or ideas on improving the content of this notebook.

Kind Regards.

Derek J. Flores R.N.

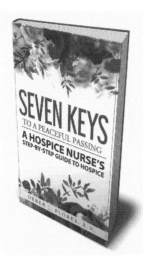

Seven Keys To Peaceful Passing is a 'Step-by-Step' Guide for patients and families to navigate their hospice journey. This easy to read book has become a standard for Hospice Nurses to share with those they care for and also for nurses themselves to review important aspects of care.

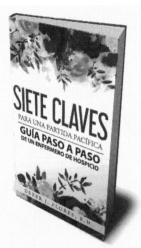

Siete Claves is the Spanish Translation of '***Seven Keys***'. The Spanish Speaking population in the U.S. is underserved in their access to comprehensive information needed to make informed decisions about Hospice Care. Please consider buying this book for your patients, it will make a real difference in outcomes.

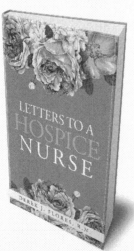

Letters to a Hospice Nurse is a collection of Love Letters written by family members left behind. This beautiful book is a wonderful way to help the healing process on the journey to find Joy again. Written for families and Hospice Team Members.

Date: Scheduled / PRN

Patient: Mileage:

Time Visit Began: Time Visit Ended:

Is pt in pain or distress?

Oriented to:

Temp: B/P: /

Resp Rate: Heart Rate:

SO2:   O2 LPM::

Pain   / 10   Last BM:

Left   MAC: Weight:
Right   MAC:

Family/Facility Updated?   Next Visit Date:

Med Supply Confirmed?

Other Notes:

Date: Scheduled / PRN

Patient: Mileage:

Time Visit Began: Time Visit Ended:

Is pt in pain or distress?

Oriented to:

Temp: B/P: /

Resp Rate: Heart Rate:

SO2: O2 LPM::

Pain   / 10 Last BM:

Left   MAC: Weight:
Right MAC:

Family/Facility Updated? Next Visit Date:

Med Supply Confirmed?

Other Notes:

Date: Scheduled / PRN

Patient: Mileage:

Time Visit Began: Time Visit Ended:

Is pt in pain or distress?

Oriented to:

Temp: B/P: /

Resp Rate: Heart Rate:

SO2:   O2 LPM::

Pain   / 10   Last BM:

Left   MAC: Weight:
Right MAC:

Family/Facility Updated?   Next Visit Date:

Med Supply Confirmed?

Other Notes:

Date: Scheduled / PRN

Patient: Mileage:

Time Visit Began: Time Visit Ended:

Is pt in pain or distress?

Oriented to:

Temp: B/P: /

Resp Rate: Heart Rate:

SO2:   O2 LPM::

Pain   / 10   Last BM:

Left   MAC: Weight:
Right MAC:

Family/Facility Updated?   Next Visit Date:

Med Supply Confirmed?

Other Notes:

Date: Scheduled / PRN

Patient: Mileage:

Time Visit Began: Time Visit Ended:

Is pt in pain or distress?

Oriented to:

Temp: B/P: /

Resp Rate: Heart Rate:

SO2:   O2 LPM::

Pain   / 10   Last BM:

Left   MAC: Weight:
Right MAC:

Family/Facility Updated?   Next Visit Date:

Med Supply Confirmed?

Other Notes:

Date: Scheduled / PRN

Patient: Mileage:

Time Visit Began: Time Visit Ended:

Is pt in pain or distress?

Oriented to:

Temp: B/P: /

Resp Rate: Heart Rate:

SO2:   O2 LPM::

Pain   / 10   Last BM:

Left   MAC: Weight:
Right MAC:

Family/Facility Updated?   Next Visit Date:

Med Supply Confirmed?

Other Notes:

Date: Scheduled / PRN

Patient: Mileage:

Time Visit Began: Time Visit Ended:

Is pt in pain or distress?

Oriented to:

Temp: B/P: /

Resp Rate: Heart Rate:

SO2:   O2 LPM::

Pain   / 10   Last BM:

Left   MAC: Weight:
Right MAC:

Family/Facility Updated?   Next Visit Date:

Med Supply Confirmed?

Other Notes:

Date: Scheduled / PRN

Patient: Mileage:

Time Visit Began: Time Visit Ended:

Is pt in pain or distress?

Oriented to:

Temp: B/P: /

Resp Rate: Heart Rate:

SO2:   O2 LPM::

Pain   / 10   Last BM:

Left   MAC: Weight:
Right MAC:

Family/Facility Updated?   Next Visit Date:

Med Supply Confirmed?

Other Notes:

Date: Scheduled / PRN

Patient: Mileage:

Time Visit Began: Time Visit Ended:

Is pt in pain or distress?

Oriented to:

Temp: B/P: /

Resp Rate: Heart Rate:

SO2:   O2 LPM::

Pain   / 10   Last BM:

Left   MAC: Weight:
Right MAC:

Family/Facility Updated?   Next Visit Date:

Med Supply Confirmed?

Other Notes:

Date: Scheduled / PRN

Patient: Mileage:

Time Visit Began: Time Visit Ended:

Is pt in pain or distress?

Oriented to:

Temp: B/P: /

Resp Rate: Heart Rate:

SO2:   O2 LPM::

Pain   / 10   Last BM:

Left   MAC: Weight:
Right   MAC:

Family/Facility Updated?   Next Visit Date:

Med Supply Confirmed?

Other Notes:

Date: Scheduled / PRN

Patient: Mileage:

Time Visit Began: Time Visit Ended:

Is pt in pain or distress?

Oriented to:

Temp: B/P: /

Resp Rate: Heart Rate:

SO2:   O2 LPM::

Pain   / 10   Last BM:

Left   MAC: Weight:
Right MAC:

Family/Facility Updated?   Next Visit Date:

Med Supply Confirmed?

Other Notes:

Date: Scheduled / PRN

Patient: Mileage:

Time Visit Began: Time Visit Ended:

Is pt in pain or distress?

Oriented to:

Temp: B/P: /

Resp Rate: Heart Rate:

SO2:   O2 LPM::

Pain   / 10   Last BM:

Left   MAC: Weight:
Right MAC:

Family/Facility Updated?   Next Visit Date:

Med Supply Confirmed?

Other Notes:

Date: Scheduled / PRN

Patient: Mileage:

Time Visit Began: Time Visit Ended:

Is pt in pain or distress?

Oriented to:

Temp: B/P: /

Resp Rate: Heart Rate:

SO2:   O2 LPM::

Pain   / 10   Last BM:

Left   MAC: Weight:
Right MAC:

Family/Facility Updated?   Next Visit Date:

Med Supply Confirmed?

Other Notes:

Date: Scheduled / PRN

Patient: Mileage:

Time Visit Began: Time Visit Ended:

Is pt in pain or distress?

Oriented to:

Temp: B/P: /

Resp Rate: Heart Rate:

SO2:   O2 LPM::

Pain   / 10   Last BM:

Left   MAC: Weight:
Right MAC:

Family/Facility Updated?   Next Visit Date:

Med Supply Confirmed?

Other Notes:

Date: Scheduled / PRN

Patient: Mileage:

Time Visit Began: Time Visit Ended:

Is pt in pain or distress?

Oriented to:

Temp: B/P: /

Resp Rate: Heart Rate:

SO2:   O2 LPM::

Pain   / 10   Last BM:

Left   MAC: Weight:
Right MAC:

Family/Facility Updated?   Next Visit Date:

Med Supply Confirmed?

Other Notes:

Date: Scheduled / PRN

Patient: Mileage:

Time Visit Began: Time Visit Ended:

Is pt in pain or distress?

Oriented to:

Temp: B/P: /

Resp Rate: Heart Rate:

SO2:   O2 LPM::

Pain   / 10   Last BM:

Left   MAC: Weight:
Right MAC:

Family/Facility Updated?   Next Visit Date:

Med Supply Confirmed?

Other Notes:

Date: Scheduled / PRN

Patient: Mileage:

Time Visit Began: Time Visit Ended:

Is pt in pain or distress?

Oriented to:

Temp: B/P: /

Resp Rate: Heart Rate:

SO2:   O2 LPM::

Pain   / 10   Last BM:

Left   MAC: Weight:
Right MAC:

Family/Facility Updated?   Next Visit Date:

Med Supply Confirmed?

Other Notes:

Date: Scheduled / PRN

Patient: Mileage:

Time Visit Began: Time Visit Ended:

Is pt in pain or distress?

Oriented to:

Temp: B/P: /

Resp Rate: Heart Rate:

SO2:   O2 LPM::

Pain   / 10   Last BM:

Left   MAC: Weight:
Right MAC:

Family/Facility Updated?   Next Visit Date:

Med Supply Confirmed?

Other Notes:

Date: Scheduled / PRN

Patient: Mileage:

Time Visit Began: Time Visit Ended:

Is pt in pain or distress?

Oriented to:

Temp: B/P: /

Resp Rate: Heart Rate:

SO2:   O2 LPM::

Pain   / 10   Last BM:

Left   MAC: Weight:
Right MAC:

Family/Facility Updated?   Next Visit Date:

Med Supply Confirmed?

Other Notes:

Date: Scheduled / PRN

Patient: Mileage:

Time Visit Began: Time Visit Ended:

Is pt in pain or distress?

Oriented to:

Temp: B/P: /

Resp Rate: Heart Rate:

SO2:   O2 LPM::

Pain   / 10   Last BM:

Left   MAC: Weight:
Right MAC:

Family/Facility Updated?   Next Visit Date:

Med Supply Confirmed?

Other Notes:

Date: Scheduled / PRN

Patient: Mileage:

Time Visit Began: Time Visit Ended:

Is pt in pain or distress?

Oriented to:

Temp: B/P: /

Resp Rate: Heart Rate:

SO2:   O2 LPM::

Pain   / 10   Last BM:

Left   MAC: Weight:
Right MAC:

Family/Facility Updated?   Next Visit Date:

Med Supply Confirmed?

Other Notes:

Date: Scheduled / PRN

Patient: Mileage:

Time Visit Began: Time Visit Ended:

Is pt in pain or distress?

Oriented to:

Temp: B/P: /

Resp Rate: Heart Rate:

SO2:   O2 LPM::

Pain   / 10   Last BM:

Left   MAC: Weight:
Right MAC:

Family/Facility Updated?   Next Visit Date:

Med Supply Confirmed?

Other Notes:

Date: Scheduled / PRN

Patient: Mileage:

Time Visit Began: Time Visit Ended:

Is pt in pain or distress?

Oriented to:

Temp: B/P: /

Resp Rate: Heart Rate:

SO2:   O2 LPM::

Pain   / 10   Last BM:

Left   MAC: Weight:
Right MAC:

Family/Facility Updated?   Next Visit Date:

Med Supply Confirmed?

Other Notes:

Date: Scheduled / PRN

Patient: Mileage:

Time Visit Began: Time Visit Ended:

Is pt in pain or distress?

Oriented to:

Temp: B/P: /

Resp Rate: Heart Rate:

SO2:   O2 LPM::

Pain   / 10   Last BM:

Left   MAC: Weight:
Right MAC:

Family/Facility Updated?   Next Visit Date:

Med Supply Confirmed?

Other Notes:

Date: Scheduled / PRN

Patient: Mileage:

Time Visit Began: Time Visit Ended:

Is pt in pain or distress?

Oriented to:

Temp: B/P: /

Resp Rate: Heart Rate:

SO2:   O2 LPM::

Pain   / 10   Last BM:

Left   MAC: Weight:
Right MAC:

Family/Facility Updated?   Next Visit Date:

Med Supply Confirmed?

Other Notes:

Date: Scheduled / PRN

Patient: Mileage:

Time Visit Began: Time Visit Ended:

Is pt in pain or distress?

Oriented to:

Temp: B/P: /

Resp Rate: Heart Rate:

SO2:   O2 LPM::

Pain   / 10   Last BM:

Left   MAC: Weight:
Right MAC:

Family/Facility Updated?   Next Visit Date:

Med Supply Confirmed?

Other Notes:

Date: Scheduled / PRN

Patient: Mileage:

Time Visit Began: Time Visit Ended:

Is pt in pain or distress?

Oriented to:

Temp: B/P: /

Resp Rate: Heart Rate:

SO2:   O2 LPM::

Pain   / 10   Last BM:

Left   MAC: Weight:
Right MAC:

Family/Facility Updated?   Next Visit Date:

Med Supply Confirmed?

Other Notes:

Date: Scheduled / PRN

Patient: Mileage:

Time Visit Began: Time Visit Ended:

Is pt in pain or distress?

Oriented to:

Temp: B/P: /

Resp Rate: Heart Rate:

SO2:   O2 LPM::

Pain   / 10   Last BM:

Left   MAC: Weight:
Right MAC:

Family/Facility Updated?   Next Visit Date:

Med Supply Confirmed?

Other Notes:

Date: Scheduled / PRN

Patient: Mileage:

Time Visit Began: Time Visit Ended:

Is pt in pain or distress?

Oriented to:

Temp: B/P: /

Resp Rate: Heart Rate:

SO2:   O2 LPM::

Pain   / 10   Last BM:

Left   MAC: Weight:
Right MAC:

Family/Facility Updated?   Next Visit Date:

Med Supply Confirmed?

Other Notes:

Date: Scheduled / PRN

Patient: Mileage:

Time Visit Began: Time Visit Ended:

Is pt in pain or distress?

Oriented to:

Temp: B/P: /

Resp Rate: Heart Rate:

SO2: O2 LPM::

Pain / 10 Last BM:

Left MAC: Weight:
Right MAC:

Family/Facility Updated? Next Visit Date:

Med Supply Confirmed?

Other Notes:

Date: Scheduled / PRN

Patient: Mileage:

Time Visit Began: Time Visit Ended:

Is pt in pain or distress?

Oriented to:

Temp: B/P: /

Resp Rate: Heart Rate:

SO2:   O2 LPM::

Pain   / 10   Last BM:

Left   MAC: Weight:
Right MAC:

Family/Facility Updated?   Next Visit Date:

Med Supply Confirmed?

Other Notes:

Date: Scheduled / PRN

Patient: Mileage:

Time Visit Began: Time Visit Ended:

Is pt in pain or distress?

Oriented to:

Temp: B/P: /

Resp Rate: Heart Rate:

SO2:   O2 LPM::

Pain   / 10   Last BM:

Left   MAC: Weight:
Right MAC:

Family/Facility Updated?   Next Visit Date:

Med Supply Confirmed?

Other Notes:

Date: Scheduled / PRN

Patient: Mileage:

Time Visit Began: Time Visit Ended:

Is pt in pain or distress?

Oriented to:

Temp: B/P: /

Resp Rate: Heart Rate:

SO2:   O2 LPM::

Pain   / 10   Last BM:

Left   MAC: Weight:
Right MAC:

Family/Facility Updated?   Next Visit Date:

Med Supply Confirmed?

Other Notes:

Date: Scheduled / PRN

Patient: Mileage:

Time Visit Began: Time Visit Ended:

Is pt in pain or distress?

Oriented to:

Temp: B/P: /

Resp Rate: Heart Rate:

SO2:   O2 LPM::

Pain   / 10   Last BM:

Left   MAC: Weight:
Right MAC:

Family/Facility Updated?   Next Visit Date:

Med Supply Confirmed?

Other Notes:

Date: Scheduled / PRN

Patient: Mileage:

Time Visit Began: Time Visit Ended:

Is pt in pain or distress?

Oriented to:

Temp: B/P: /

Resp Rate: Heart Rate:

SO2:   O2 LPM::

Pain   / 10   Last BM:

Left   MAC: Weight:
Right MAC:

Family/Facility Updated?   Next Visit Date:

Med Supply Confirmed?

Other Notes:

Date: Scheduled / PRN

Patient: Mileage:

Time Visit Began: Time Visit Ended:

Is pt in pain or distress?

Oriented to:

Temp: B/P: /

Resp Rate: Heart Rate:

SO2:   O2 LPM::

Pain   / 10   Last BM:

Left   MAC: Weight:
Right MAC:

Family/Facility Updated?   Next Visit Date:

Med Supply Confirmed?

Other Notes:

Date: Scheduled / PRN

Patient: Mileage:

Time Visit Began: Time Visit Ended:

Is pt in pain or distress?

Oriented to:

Temp: B/P: /

Resp Rate: Heart Rate:

SO2:   O2 LPM::

Pain   / 10   Last BM:

Left   MAC: Weight:
Right MAC:

Family/Facility Updated?   Next Visit Date:

Med Supply Confirmed?

Other Notes:

Date: Scheduled / PRN

Patient: Mileage:

Time Visit Began: Time Visit Ended:

Is pt in pain or distress?

Oriented to:

Temp: B/P: /

Resp Rate: Heart Rate:

SO2:   O2 LPM::

Pain   / 10   Last BM:

Left   MAC: Weight:
Right MAC:

Family/Facility Updated?   Next Visit Date:

Med Supply Confirmed?

Other Notes:

Date: Scheduled / PRN

Patient: Mileage:

Time Visit Began: Time Visit Ended:

Is pt in pain or distress?

Oriented to:

Temp: B/P: /

Resp Rate: Heart Rate:

SO2: O2 LPM::

Pain / 10 Last BM:

Left MAC: Weight:
Right MAC:

Family/Facility Updated? Next Visit Date:

Med Supply Confirmed?

Other Notes:

Date: Scheduled / PRN

Patient: Mileage:

Time Visit Began: Time Visit Ended:

Is pt in pain or distress?

Oriented to:

Temp: B/P: /

Resp Rate: Heart Rate:

SO2:   O2 LPM::

Pain   / 10   Last BM:

Left   MAC: Weight:
Right MAC:

Family/Facility Updated?   Next Visit Date:

Med Supply Confirmed?

Other Notes:

Date: Scheduled / PRN

Patient: Mileage:

Time Visit Began: Time Visit Ended:

Is pt in pain or distress?

Oriented to:

Temp: B/P: /

Resp Rate: Heart Rate:

SO2: O2 LPM::

Pain / 10 Last BM:

Left   MAC: Weight:
Right MAC:

Family/Facility Updated? Next Visit Date:

Med Supply Confirmed?

Other Notes:

Date: Scheduled / PRN

Patient: Mileage:

Time Visit Began: Time Visit Ended:

Is pt in pain or distress?

Oriented to:

Temp: B/P: /

Resp Rate: Heart Rate:

SO2:   O2 LPM::

Pain   / 10   Last BM:

Left   MAC: Weight:
Right MAC:

Family/Facility Updated?   Next Visit Date:

Med Supply Confirmed?

Other Notes:

Date: Scheduled / PRN

Patient: Mileage:

Time Visit Began: Time Visit Ended:

Is pt in pain or distress?

Oriented to:

Temp: B/P: /

Resp Rate: Heart Rate:

SO2:   O2 LPM::

Pain   / 10   Last BM:

Left   MAC: Weight:
Right MAC:

Family/Facility Updated?   Next Visit Date:

Med Supply Confirmed?

Other Notes:

Date: Scheduled / PRN

Patient: Mileage:

Time Visit Began: Time Visit Ended:

Is pt in pain or distress?

Oriented to:

Temp: B/P: /

Resp Rate: Heart Rate:

SO2:   O2 LPM::

Pain   / 10   Last BM:

Left   MAC: Weight:
Right MAC:

Family/Facility Updated?   Next Visit Date:

Med Supply Confirmed?

Other Notes:

Date: Scheduled / PRN

Patient: Mileage:

Time Visit Began: Time Visit Ended:

Is pt in pain or distress?

Oriented to:

Temp: B/P: /

Resp Rate: Heart Rate:

SO2:   O2 LPM::

Pain   / 10   Last BM:

Left   MAC: Weight:
Right MAC:

Family/Facility Updated?   Next Visit Date:

Med Supply Confirmed?

Other Notes:

Date: Scheduled / PRN

Patient: Mileage:

Time Visit Began: Time Visit Ended:

Is pt in pain or distress?

Oriented to:

Temp: B/P: /

Resp Rate: Heart Rate:

SO2:   O2 LPM::

Pain   / 10   Last BM:

Left   MAC: Weight:
Right MAC:

Family/Facility Updated?   Next Visit Date:

Med Supply Confirmed?

Other Notes:

Date: Scheduled / PRN

Patient: Mileage:

Time Visit Began: Time Visit Ended:

Is pt in pain or distress?

Oriented to:

Temp: B/P: /

Resp Rate: Heart Rate:

SO2:   O2 LPM::

Pain   / 10   Last BM:

Left   MAC: Weight:
Right MAC:

Family/Facility Updated?   Next Visit Date:

Med Supply Confirmed?

Other Notes:

Date: Scheduled / PRN

Patient: Mileage:

Time Visit Began: Time Visit Ended:

Is pt in pain or distress?

Oriented to:

Temp: B/P: /

Resp Rate: Heart Rate:

SO2:   O2 LPM::

Pain   / 10   Last BM:

Left   MAC: Weight:
Right MAC:

Family/Facility Updated?   Next Visit Date:

Med Supply Confirmed?

Other Notes:

Date: Scheduled / PRN

Patient: Mileage:

Time Visit Began: Time Visit Ended:

Is pt in pain or distress?

Oriented to:

Temp: B/P: /

Resp Rate: Heart Rate:

SO2:   O2 LPM::

Pain   / 10   Last BM:

Left   MAC: Weight:
Right MAC:

Family/Facility Updated?   Next Visit Date:

Med Supply Confirmed?

Other Notes:

Date: Scheduled / PRN

Patient: Mileage:

Time Visit Began: Time Visit Ended:

Is pt in pain or distress?

Oriented to:

Temp: B/P: /

Resp Rate: Heart Rate:

SO2:   O2 LPM::

Pain   / 10   Last BM:

Left   MAC: Weight:
Right MAC:

Family/Facility Updated?   Next Visit Date:

Med Supply Confirmed?

Other Notes:

Date: Scheduled / PRN

Patient: Mileage:

Time Visit Began: Time Visit Ended:

Is pt in pain or distress?

Oriented to:

Temp: B/P: /

Resp Rate: Heart Rate:

SO2: O2 LPM::

Pain / 10 Last BM:

Left   MAC: Weight:
Right MAC:

Family/Facility Updated? Next Visit Date:

Med Supply Confirmed?

Other Notes:

Date: Scheduled / PRN

Patient: Mileage:

Time Visit Began: Time Visit Ended:

Is pt in pain or distress?

Oriented to:

Temp: B/P: /

Resp Rate: Heart Rate:

SO2:   O2 LPM::

Pain   / 10   Last BM:

Left   MAC: Weight:
Right MAC:

Family/Facility Updated?   Next Visit Date:

Med Supply Confirmed?

Other Notes:

Date: Scheduled / PRN

Patient: Mileage:

Time Visit Began: Time Visit Ended:

Is pt in pain or distress?

Oriented to:

Temp: B/P: /

Resp Rate: Heart Rate:

SO2: O2 LPM::

Pain / 10 Last BM:

Left MAC: Weight:
Right MAC:

Family/Facility Updated? Next Visit Date:

Med Supply Confirmed?

Other Notes:

Made in the USA
Las Vegas, NV
17 May 2021

23187321R00063